HERBAL MEDICINE FOR CHILDREN

by Frances Hambly

Published by
Amberwood Publishing Ltd
Rochester, England

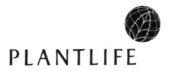

PLANTLIFE

Registered Charity No. 328576

Amberwood Publishing supports the Plantlife Charity, Britain's only charity exclusively dedicated to saving wild plants.

ISBN 1-899308-30-X

Cover design by Studio Read

Printed in Great Britain

CONTENTS

About the Author

Frances Hambly has been a practising medical herbalist since 1987 and is a member of the National Institute of Medical Herbalists. She later studied Aromatic Medicine with Dr Daniel Penoel.

She has been a student mentor, examiner and a post graduate lecturer for the NIMH. She practices in East Sussex where she and her husband run a successful clinic and herbal dispensary.

Frances had a fascination for medicine and plants from a young age as she was brought up using herbs which came from the garden or products from her family in Switzerland. This led on to her knowing that she wanted to become a herbalist. With two children of her own she is committed to natural ways of raising children and treating childhood illnesses.

She offers prenatal advice on conception, pregnancy and childbirth and gives regular talks to postnatal groups on herbs, nutrition and vaccination.

Her first book *Herbalism* was co-written with her husband Paul Hambly.

Acknowledgements

My thanks to my colleagues David Caudwell and Lucy Vertue for proof-reading and advice, to June Crisp at Amberwood, and to my family, Paul for his help and support and Eleanor and Finn for teaching me so much.

Note to Reader

Whilst the author has made every effort to ensure that the contents of this book are accurate in every particular, it is not intended to be regarded as a substitute for professional medical advice under treatment. Readers are urged to give careful consideration to any difficulties which they may be experiencing with their own health and to consult their General Practitioner if uncertain as to its cause or nature. Neither the author nor the publisher can accept any legal responsibility for any health problem which results from use of the self-help methods described.

Foreword

In times like these when parents are thirsty for knowledge of how they can best care for their children and keep them in optimum health, a book such as this is very welcome. We are not taught formally about child care at school or university, but with education provided by books such as Frances', combined with innate parental instinct, we can go a long way to ensure that we provide the right ingredients for our children's health and well being. Furthermore, we can ensure that we have the right tools at the ready to aid our children bounce back to health when ill.

We all have self healing mechanisms that are continually enabling us to maintain health and balance which are enhanced by healthy diet and lifestyle. When we succumb to infection and illness we can use foods and herbs to aid the healing process and speed recovery. Frances' book provides a simple, easy to understand, guide to the recognition of common childhood illnesses and clear concise instructions for treating these with herbs. Such information can enable parents to incorporate herbs into their everyday life with confidence and thus use the raw ingredients around them to treat common self limiting illness at home and minimise visits to the doctor and administration of medicines such as antibiotics.

Most parents know when their children are off-colour and in the prodromal stage of illness and for this reason they are in the best position to administer treatment to their children and resolve the symptoms quickly. The right foods and herbs combined with caring and nurturing home nursing will frequently see the symptoms off before they really set in. Frances' long experience with herbs as a practising herbalist and a mother, which comes through in the clear and authoritative way that she writes, encapsulated in the format of this easy reference alphabetical guide, will provide help and support for parents as they care for their children and is definitely recommended as one they should have on their bookshelves.

Anne McIntyre FNIMH

1 | Introduction

The aim of this book is to provide a reference for recognising a range of typical childhood problems and treating them with herbs. It can also be used as a guide as to how to keep children healthy. The format is alphabetical, giving a description of the condition, followed by advice on when to seek professional help, diet and herbs.

Instructions as to how to prepare the herbs and how to administer them including dosage are given at the beginning of the book in *Using Herbs with Children*.

All the herbs given in the book are safe, gentle and effective for children. If a condition does not resolve itself quickly it is always best to seek professional help. It is not worth delaying treatment if you are unsure of anything. There are stronger herbs that might be used in more severe cases of illness but these need to be prescribed by a qualified Herbalist.

2 | How to view disease

Seeing a sick child can be as distressing for the parent as it is for the child. The wish to alleviate the suffering as quickly as possible is only normal; however, the administration of powerful drugs such as antibiotics, steroids and sedatives can have long-term repercussions. There is a place for the latter, one wouldn't question the use of antibiotics in meningitis, but too often they are considered as the only treatment available. Children have an innate ability to bounce back to health and they respond remarkably well to herbal medicines. More often than not a gentle herbal remedy will be more effective than a powerful drug. Antibiotics destroy the body's normal ecology of bacteria that protect us. Steroids suppress inflammation which is part of the healing process. Strong sedatives dull the vitality and ability of the child to function fully.

It helps to regard childhood illnesses as stages in their development, so often a child has noticeably strengthened physically and mentally progressed after being ill. Chinese medicine sees childhood diseases as a result of toxins accumulated while in the womb and they are viewed as a cleansing process.

A fever should be regarded as the response of a healthy body, it is Nature's way of ridding the body of toxins and should not be unnecessarily impeded by way of administering paracetomol. It is of course important to keep a careful eye on the progress of a fever; especially in young children whose temperature regulation is still not fully developed. Much can be done herbally and with water to check a fever without impinging on its positive effects.

Fundamental to a child's ability to avoid, cope with, and rid itself of disease is good housing, clean water, a healthy diet, fresh air and exercise and a loving secure environment. This is what we continually strive to give our children as they grow up, it is not something that comes off the shelf.

Emotional upsets and feeling unloved can be a cause of illness. Some children become ill because they don't get enough attention or are particularly needy – a cry for love.

We live in a busy world and illness can be very inconvenient with the pressures of school and work on parents. However, it is important to recognise the first signs of illness and allow children to recover properly. Thankfully children tend to bounce back quickly, if they don't the cause needs to be addressed. Most parents recognise when a child isn't 100%, this is the time to start keeping things quiet, skip social and after school activities and get them to bed early.

Limit television and computer games. Rest (physical and mental) and good nutrition are vital. Keep this going after the acute phase of illness is over and combine with fresh air and some exercise. Convalescence is something we think of for the elderly but everybody needs time to recover and regenerate after an illness.

Our knowledge of how to nurse a sick child has been somewhat eroded over the generations and led to a lack of confidence when dealing with illness.

A bout of illness can be a special time to nurture and bond with your child and discover your own innate nursing abilities.

3 | The immune system

The immune system is vital to good health, protecting the body from organisms and clearing up the debris from the bodily processes.

The effectiveness of the immune system can be compromised by a number of things – antibiotics, steroids, a bad diet, pollution, stress, emotional distress and inherited factors. If the immune system is compromised, infections such as colds can be continual.

The blood contains cells to attack and destroy organisms, but if the infection is more severe the lymphatic system comes into play. This is the network of tiny vessels which carry the lymph fluid. The lymph picks up the debris and microbes and carries them via the vessels to the lymph nodes which are some of the main sites of immune activity in the body. The lymph nodes are situated in groups called lymph glands. They contain large numbers of white blood cells and enlarge as the cells multiply when the body is under attack. They literally eat up the invading organisms. In a highly infectious disease, antibodies are produced against the organism to protect the body from reinfection in the future. The debris resulting from the infection is carried to the liver to be detoxified and excreted. The liver, spleen, lining of the digestive system, tonsils and adenoids all contain lymphatic tissue. The lymph glands are most easily palpable in the neck along the line of the jaw from under the ears.

A healthy diet is vital for a healthy immune system, see page 13. Herbs like Echinacea can be taken to boost the function of the immune system.

Exercise activates what is called the lymphatic pump which improves the circulation of lymph around the body.

A good immune system is able to deal quickly and effectively with invading organisms. A weakness in the body, eg poor digestion leading to poor nutritional uptake, will put a strain on the immune system and weaken it because it isn't receiving enough of the essential nutrients for it to function 100%.

Auto-immune disease occurs when the immune system starts to attack the body's own tissues. When this occurs, the control mechanism which normally stops invading organisms has broken down.

Vaccination

Viewing disease as a positive part of childhood brings up the vexed question of vaccination. Whether to vaccinate your child or not is an extremely difficult decision to make. It is important to be aware of all the facts in order to make an informed choice. This can be rather overwhelming in the initial weeks of your baby's life, and most of us are too focussed on the birth to think about vaccinations before baby's arrival. Talk to several different practitioners and read as much literature as possible on the subject to make the decision you are most comfortable with. It is important that whatever your decision you have the support of a practitioner who will be available when your child is ill and you need advice.

If there is a family history of allergies, asthma, eczema or febrile convulsions it is worth being extremely cautious before proceeding with vaccinations.

It is important to strengthen your child's immune system whatever your choice and make sure your child is 100% well on the day of any vaccinations.

Around the time of a vaccination supplement with a good quality children's vitamin and mineral supplement and cold-pressed oils.

How children will react to a vaccine is unpredictable. Evidence suggests certain blood groups cope better than others. Herbs and Homoeopathy can be used to minimise side effects, alongside Acupuncture and Cranial osteopathy to help more long-term problems.

Herbalists have traditionally used herbs like Hyssop to strengthen the immune system and limit the effect of diseases like whooping cough.

It is necessary to look at whether vaccination actually prevents disease. It does not guarantee that your child will not get the disease and there is evidence connecting vaccination to chronic conditions like asthma and eczema and auto-immune diseases like arthritis, and bowel disorders and ME.

4 | Signs of illness

It is important to respond quickly to the first signs of illness in a child before waiting to see what happens. Most childhood illnesses are self-limiting, but it is still better to act preventatively through diet and herbs and making sure your child has enough rest. For example, Whooping cough (see below) is virtually impossible to diagnose until the whoop starts, when treatment is difficult. Boosting your child's immune system, removing sugary foods from their diet and restricting cow's milk, not letting them get over-excited or become over-tired and treating colds and coughs as they manifest, can do much to avert the degree of illness and prevent complications. Most parents know when something is not quite right with their child.

Initial signs of illness include:
- Poor appetite.
- Sleeping more.
- Lethargic and quiet.
- Restless and irritable.
- Disturbed nights.
- Change from normal behaviour.
- Crying for no apparent reason.

Warning signs

The following need immediate emergency treatment:
- Dehydration – not passed water for 24 hours, sunken eyes.
- Listless, silent.
- Heaving chest and flaring nostrils.
- Diarrhoea and vomiting – if more than 6 hours in babies.
- Sensitivity to light (photophobia), stiff neck, (purpuric) rash.

5 | Diet during childhood

Food is fundamental to a child's well-being and of paramount importance in building a healthy immune system. The recipe for a healthy child lies in the food he or she eats! Choose fresh organic foods wherever possible.

In the first year of life milk is the most important food for a baby and breast milk is all they require nutritionally for the first six months. Cow's milk formula can cause problems with a baby's digestive system and skin sensitivities like eczema. Goat's milk formula is an alternative in these situations.

Weaning

This can be critical for a child's immune system and future development. If there is any history of allergy in the family special care needs to be taken. The majority of commercially produced baby foods and drinks contain sugar, which is completely unnecessary and taints a baby's palate for the future. It can also cause hypersensitivity, making your child irritable, fractious and lead to sleep problems and hyperactivity.

Dairy products, wheat, eggs and oranges are among the most common allergenic foods. Too early exposure to these can set up a sensitivity to them. It is worth not introducing these into your baby's diet until they are 10-12 months old, especially if there is an allergic family history. Again, many commercial baby foods will contain these foods, so it is important to read the label carefully.

Meat is not necessary when children are very young, and they might find it difficult to digest and constipating.

When first introducing solid foods give only one food at a time, so that if there is a reaction you know what is causing it. Sensitivity to a food can cause colic, diarrhoea, irritability, catarrh or a skin rash. If there is a reaction wait at least a month before introducing it again. Ideal foods to introduce are pureed carrot, pear or apple, followed by a wider variety of vegetables, fruit and baby rice. Avoid any foods that you or your partner are sensitive to until later, along with wheat etc. Introduce one new food a week.

Make sure your child is not over-excited or too tired to eat. Be relaxed and don't worry about them making a mess !

Make sure they are having enough fluid when going onto solids as there is a tendency towards constipation as a baby's digestive system adjusts to the change from a liquid diet.

Appetite

Children's appetites vary widely from one child to another. They can also vary from day to day with fads for certain foods coming and going. For example, your child might eat bananas every day for several weeks, then not touch another one for a month. Children have a strong sense of what they need and fulfil their nutritional requirements by eating in this way. They can also get bored with the same foods. It is self-defeating to force children to eat what they don't like, but keep introducing a small amount of these and new foods for them to try. However, a child's natural instinct for what's good for him or her can be destroyed by inappropriate weaning and a diet with too much sugar, salt and processed foods.

Vital nutrients

VITAMINS

Vitamin A
- for resistance to infections, growth and repair, healthy eyes, gums and skin.
- from fish, organic liver, cheese, green and orange vegetables (carrots), salads, eggs, butter.

B vitamins
- for a healthy nervous system and metabolism, and red blood cell formation.
- from bread, milk, meat, yeast extract, green veg, fish, eggs, cereal, rice, yoghurt, soya, beans.

Vitamin C

- for protection from viruses and toxins, enhances iron absorption, aids healing.
- from fresh fruit and vegetables.

Vitamin D

- for normal bone and teeth formation and growth.
- from oily fish like sardines, liver, dairy, sunlight.

Vitamin E

- for essential fatty acid metabolism and red blood cell manufacture.
- from eggs, bread, butter, wholewheat, green vegetables, sunflower oil, cereals, peanut butter.

MINERALS

Calcium

- for healthy bones and teeth along with Magnesium.
- from cheese, yoghurt, milk, nuts (especially almonds), beans, green vegetables, soya products (tofu), seeds, tahini (sesame seed paste), figs, tinned salmon and sardines, cereals (oatmeal).

Magnesium

- vital to bone and teeth formation, and nerve and muscle function.
- from green vegetables, beans, nuts and seeds, wholegrains, seafood, eggs.

Iron

- for haemoglobin production, vital to oxygen transport in the blood.
- from wholegrains, green vegetables, meat, egg yolk, molasses.

Zinc

- vital to the efficient functioning of the immune system, involved in wound healing and tissue repair.
- from nuts and seeds (eg pumpkin), yeast, eggs, fruit and vegetables, meat, shellfish.

Protein

Eggs, fish, meat, milk products, poultry and soya beans are all complete proteins – containing all the essential amino acids. Good sources of non-animal protein, other than soya, are derived from grains, pulses, nuts and seeds. Vegetable proteins (except soya) are incomplete proteins and need to be eaten in combination, for example: rice, nuts and greens.

Try to choose organic animal produce which hasn't been subject to intensive farming techniques. Antibiotics, growth hormones etc can have a negative and long-term effect on the health of our children. Avoid fish from fish farms unless organic. Fish with skins, and shellfish, which are scavengers tend to live in polluted estuaries and shallow waters. Fish also tend to accumulate mercury.

Animal protein does not need to be eaten to excess, a small quantity of more expensive meat is far healthier. Too much animal protein can contribute to constipation.

Try to buy nuts in their shells and dry roast them at home. Commercial nut butters are often made with hydrogenated oil and easily become rancid. Look for unhydrogenated nut butters made with unhydrogenated fats.

Essential fatty acids

These nutrients are vital to the functioning of the immune system and the maintenance of the nervous and hormonal system, and healthy skin. They are involved with the formation of every cell membrane in the body.

The body is unable to manufacture these essential fatty acids (EFA's) and has to obtain them from the diet. There are two main groups of EFAs: Omega-3 and Omega-6. Omega-6 EFAs are found mainly in seeds like safflower, sunflower and pumpkin seeds, and evening primrose oil. Omega-3 oils are obtained from linseed (flax) oil, walnut and wheatgerm oil, as well as from fresh oily fish like salmon, sardines and tuna.

EFAs are also found in green vegetables, wheat and beans, including soya. Heat, light, cooking and processing will destroy EFAs, so they need to be obtained from fresh foods.

Oils from nuts and seeds need to be cold-pressed. They can be used in yoghurt, desserts, shakes, mayonnaise or salad dressings. If there are skin problems include Borage or Hempseed oil in the diet. Alternatively, supplement with a blend of Omega-3 and 6 EFAs.

Use butter in moderation and/or an unhydrogenated margarine for spreading. Hydrogenated fats and oils are best avoided due to their toxic nature. Cold-pressed olive oil is a good oil to include in the daily diet and is the best oil for cooking.

Our diets today tend to be very low in EFAs and high in harmful fats. We tend to see all fat as bad and think low fat is best. It is vital for childrens' growth and development to have the full complement of healthy fats. Most commercial oils are heat extracted, refined and hydrogenated which destroys the EFAs and makes them nutritionally inferior, if not toxic by nature. These oils release damaging free radicals into the blood.

Dairy products

Milk is specifically designed for the developing young, in the case of cow's milk for the growing calf. Cow's milk formula produces quite a different gut flora to breast milk in babies. In humans the ability to digest milk is extended all the time it is consumed. An enzyme in the stomach called lactase allows humans to digest milk sugar (lactose). Lactase ceases to be produced in early childhood in two thirds of the world population. Only a third of the world's population inherit the ability to digest lactose after weaning. Undigested lactose accumulates and irritates the bowel causing bloating, wind and discomfort. Diarrhoea and gut infections like gastroenteritis can cause temporary lactose intolerance.

Some children are allergic to the proteins in milk, these are the curds (casein) and whey (beta-lactoglobulin). This can manifest as eczema, asthma, respiratory or digestive disturbances. Intolerance to milk protein can be hereditary or due to too early an introduction of cow's milk into the diet, the large protein molecules sensitising the digestive system.

The first question asked when restricting the amount of dairy foods in the diet is always about calcium. It is obviously important to maintain enough calcium in the diet of a growing child. However, if a child is being compromised by dairy products they might well be being deprived of enough nutrients anyway. Breast milk is in fact a relatively low source of calcium which helps to put things in perspective as regards requirements.

It is rare to be intolerant to the lactose and proteins of all types of dairy products. Yoghurt is usually well tolerated by those with an intolerance to lactose or milk protein. If there is a major intolerance to cow's milk choose goat or sheep's yoghurt instead.

The bacteria that make live yoghurt produce enzymes that convert lactose into lactic acid and break the protein molecules (the curds and whey) into smaller components that do not aggravate the digestive system. Live yoghurt promotes a healthy gut flora and is a good source of calcium.

There is a threshold level of tolerance to lactose before it causes problems. Most hard cheeses – cheddar, edam, gouda contain low levels of lactose and butter contains very little. Milk (especially low fat), cream and cream/soft cheeses contain the most lactose. Cultured products like creme fraiche, greek yoghurt and quark are alternatives. All dairy products are a relatively poor source of magnesium and magnesium rich foods need to be included in the diet to ensure healthy bones.

If all milk products need to be avoided see above for the other sources of calcium. Alternatives to cow's milk include soya milk, yoghurt and ice cream, rice or oat milk. Apple or grape juice instead of milk on cereal can be quite palatable.

Salt

Processed food and ready meals are packed with high levels of hidden salt so beware.

Use minimum quantities of salt in cooking and preferably choose an unrefined sea salt (Atlantic/Celtic salt) which is greyish in colour and does not contain additives to make it free flowing. It is a good source of minerals. When adding salt to a meal encourage the use of a herb salt.

Too much salt puts a strain on the kidneys and leads to problems in later life like arteriosclerosis, water retention and high blood pressure.

Sugar

Sugar is incorporated into so many food products it is difficult to avoid without reading food and drink labels. Children's palates quickly desire the sweeter taste. Apart from causing tooth decay, sugar can cause hyperactivity, irritability and mood swings in children as well as depressing the immune system.

Sugar is widely used in commercial cereals, processed and tinned foods, cakes, biscuits, ice cream, chocolate, jams, sweets and fizzy drinks.

White sugar is devoid of all nutrients, supplying only calories, while robbing the body of precious vitamins and minerals. Demerara sugar in moderation is better than refined white sugar, supplying some nutrients, with molasses providing a good source of vitamins and minerals, like iron. Alternative sweeteners to sugar include real maple syrup, date syrup, pear and apple spread, honey, sugar-free jams made with concentrated juices, dried fruit and sweet ripe fruit like bananas and dates. Instead of sugary, fizzy drinks use concentrated fruit juices diluted with water.

Wheat

Wheat tends to be part of the staple diet, but it can also become a common food allergen. Ideally it should not be introduced into a baby's diet until 10-12 months old.

Wheat can cause digestive and mental disturbances in sensitive individuals, and since wheat is a grass it can aggravate the symptoms of hay fever.

Although too many wholemeal products are not good for young children, wholemeal bread is generally considered healthier for older children. However, unless this is organic this might mean increasing their consumption of pesticides. Wholemeal uses the wholegrain, this includes the outside husk which contains the highest levels of pesticide residue. Indeed, it may well be the pesticides rather than the wheat causing problems. If buying wholemeal flour, bread and pasta choose organic. Organic wheat is also likely to be higher in nutrients such as selenium and silica.

It is worth checking the amount of wheat in your child's diet and provide variety with rice, oats and rye in cereals, biscuits, crackers, breads and snacks. Spelt flour is an ancient wheat that is generally better tolerated by those who are sensitive to wheat.

Diet During Infections

During any acute illness keep children on a light diet. Most children lose their appetite anyway, don't force them to eat, it will only put more strain on the system. If there is a fever just give plenty of fluids such as pure water, herb teas, diluted fruit juices. Don't give any dairy produce, especially with any catarrhal conditions of the respiratory tract or stomach. When the acute stage is over give plenty of fruit and vegetables. Vegetable soup or chicken broth are ideal. Beetroot juice can be given diluted with water and carrot or apple juice to boost the immune system. Garlic can be included in juices and soups, preferably raw, where it can be crushed and added last thing. Alternatively, halve a piece of garlic and rub this on the soles of each foot.

Useful supplements during and after an infection include Floradix, Kindervital and Vitamin C with bioflavonoids and rosehips.

6 | Pollution in our environment

We are surrounded by all sorts of pollution, from the residue of pesticides in food and traffic fumes to electromagnetic and noise pollution. In the home, furniture, bedding, flooring and even clothes can give off vapours from the glues used during manufacture and installation and fabric treatments like fire retardants. Solvent-based paints (gloss), varnishes and glues used while decorating give off powerful fumes.

Household cleaners, air fresheners, cigarette smoke, insect repellents and garden chemicals are further hazards. Some of these chemicals have been linked with a higher incidence of childhood leukaemia and other illnesses.

Allergies are being connected to being brought up in too sterile an environment, so exposure to a bit of dirt is healthier than disinfecting every surface.

Obviously, it is impossible to avoid exposure to all chemicals but we can limit what our children are exposed to by creating a healthy home and choosing environmentally and people-friendly products. Using anti-radiation computer screens, limiting television exposure, switching electrical appliances off in the bedroom at night and having windows open as much as possible all have a positive effect on creating a healthier environment.

Some children will be more susceptible to developing allergies and chemical sensitivities, the risk can be reduced by limiting the threshold level of exposure.

7 | Using herbs with children

Herbs can be used very effectively as the first line of treatment. Herbal Medicine is wonderfully versatile and does not have to be the concoction of foul-tasting remedies often conjured up in the imagination! Herbs can be administered as poultices, linaments, hand and footbaths, as well as in the bath, eardrops, nosedrops, ointments, capsules or tablets, drops, sprays, and teas and syrups that are soothing and pleasant to take.

Seeing a herbalist

It is a wise idea to get to know a qualified Herbalist in your area who suits your needs as a family. Always choose a qualified Herbalist with the letters MNIMH, FNIMH or CPP after their name. There is nothing to replace a consultation, where the practitioner can get to know you and your child/ren. Suggestions can be made as to diet and any supplements and which herbs you should have on hand. This makes it possible to deal with queries over the phone and allows for short follow-up consultations when required. Find out what happens when your practitioner is on holiday and what sort of cover is provided.

Where to get your herbs

Your Herbalist or a specialist herbal dispensary run by qualified Herbalists and with trained staff is undoubtedly the most reliable place to obtain your herbs. The quality will be good and you will receive professional advice and the correct dosage regimes. With essential oils it is vital that they are pure and labelled correctly.

How to use herbs with children

Infusions/teas
These are made using the leaves and/or flowers of the fresh or dried herb. Place 1 tsp of the the dried or 2 tsp of the fresh herb into a teapot and

pour on a cup of boiling water, cover and leave to brew for 5-10 minutes. For babies use ½ tsp herb per cup of liquid or ½ of a cup of adult dose diluted and given 2-4 times a day.

Herb teas can be drunk quite freely and intake is naturally limited by the quantity of fluid. As a guide, ½ a cup 2-4 times a day for 2-6 years old and 1 cup 2-4 times a day over 6 years old. Teas can be mixed with water or juice and sipped hot or cold over the day.

Decoctions

These are made using the woodier parts of the herbs – roots, bark and seeds – which need to be simmered to extract the active ingredients. The material should be cut or crushed into small pieces to allow for the best extraction, a pestle and mortar or coffee grinder are ideal for this. Place 1-2 tsp into a stainless steel, enamelled or glass saucepan with a lid, not aluminium. Add 2-3 cups of water and simmer for 10-15 minutes. These will be rather strong for children to take and are probably best administerd in baths.

Baths

These are an excellent way of administering herbs to babies and young children since the skin is a very good medium through which to absorb herbs into the system.

Use 50g of dried herbs or 100g of fresh per 1 litre of boiled water. Infuse for 10-15 minutes in a covered vessel. Strain through a tea strainer or muslin into a shallow bath. The residual herbal material can be infused again with another litre of boiled water and added to the bath to make it stronger, or kept covered and used the next day. For bark and roots make up as a decoction. Alternatively, pour the tea into a china, glass or enamelled bowl and immerse the feet or hands in the water for 8-10 minutes. *Hand and Footbaths* are more suitable for older children.

Eyebaths – simmer the herbs for 1-2 minutes to achieve sterility, then strain through a piece of muslin or a coffee filter. The addition of a few grains of sea salt to the eyebath is helpful. Alternatively, add 1-3 drops of tincture to an eyebathful of boiled or distilled water.

Compress

This is simply a muslin, flannel or piece of cotton wool soaked in an infusion, decoction or tincture of the appropriate herb/s and then applied to the affected area for 5-10 minutes. It can be used cold or hot.

Poultice

The herbs are placed in a cotton bag or muslin and applied to the affected area. Use 2-4 tablespoons of the mixture of dried herbs and mix with an equal amount of slippery elm or rolled oats and place in the bag. Place in a bowl and slowly pour on boiling water until the contents are wet. Leave for 5-10 minutes and apply while warm. Leave it in place for 5-15 minutes.

Syrups

A syrup is simple to make by slicing an onion and putting it at the bottom of a glass jar and covering it with honey or brown sugar. Put the lid on and leave in a warm place overnight and then strain and store in an airtight container. Medicinal in itself it is also a good way to disguise the taste of stronger medicines.

Dosages for Children

Tinctures

While a baby is being solely breast-fed, the mother can take the full adult dose which will come through the milk to the baby. The standard adult dose is 5mls three times a day. Generally speaking, children of 12 years and over can take the full adult dose, children 6 years and over half the adult dose, children over 2 years a third of the adult dose and babies a tenth. However, herbs work well as drops and this allows for a more tailored dosage system which can easily be administrated in a little water or juice.

FOR BABIES

0-6 months	1-5 drops
6-12 months	5-10 drops
12-24 months	10-15 drops

FOR CHILDREN

2-5 years	20-40 drops (0.5-1ml)
5-12 years	1.5-2.5ml (½ tsp)

Essential oils

FOR ADDING TO THE BATH:

Babies: 2-3 drops in the bath. This can be added to a few ml of dispersant first.
2 year olds 5 drops per bath.

WHEN MAKING UP AN OIL TO APPLY TO THE SKIN:

1 drop of essential oil in 5ml of base oil (eg Almond oil) for babies.
1 drop in 2.5ml for children over 2 years old.

8 | An A–Z of childhood illnesses

ADENOIDS

The adenoids are part of the immune system. They swell when the body is fighting an infection or there is an allergic reaction. When inflamed and enlarged they interfere with breathing, making the speech sound nasal and causing congestion in the eustachian tubes. This in turn increases the susceptibility to ear infections and interference with hearing. See also *Earache* and *Tonsilitis*.

WHEN TO SEEK PROFESSIONAL HELP

- If it is a recurring problem.

DIET AND SUPPLEMENTS

- See *Diet during infections* on page 19.
- A food intolerance or allergy is often the suspect, in particular cow's milk.

HERBS

- Cleavers and Marigold are wonderful lymphatic tonics and can be taken plentifully.
- Echinacea will boost the immune system.

ATTENTION DEFICIT DISORDER(ADD), AUTISM

These need specialised help and need to be treated multifactorially. See *Allergies, Anxiety, Hyperactivity*.

ALLERGIES

These are caused when the body's immune system reacts to internal or external substances that are not necessarily harmful to the body.

Food allergies can often be traced back to the introduction of dairy produce or wheat at too early an age. It is advisable not to introduce the most allergenic foods such as cow's milk and wheat too early into a baby's diet.

Breast-feeding helps to boost a baby's immune system and reduce the risk of allergy, although with a sensitive individual and where there is a genetic disposition, certain food substances can pass through the breast milk and sensitise the baby.

Allergies can present in many ways – as skin reactions like eczema, as respiratory problems like asthma, sneezing, a constant stuffy or runny nose, as digestive symptoms such as diarrhoea, constipation and stomach pain, as well as headaches, lethargy, hyperactivity and sleeplessness.

If dietary changes and herbs don't work the problem might be candidiasis. See also *Asthma, Candida/Candidiasis* and *Eczema*.

WHEN TO SEEK PROFESSIONAL HELP

- Due to the complex nature of allergies it is advisable to work in conjunction with a practitioner, especially when embarking on a restricted diet.

DIET AND SUPPLEMENTS

- Choose organic foods where possible and cut out junk and processed foods, additives and refined sugar.
- Include cold-pressed oils in the child's diet.
- Balance the amount of any one food in the day, eg limit wheat to once a day.
- See *Diet during Childhood* on page 13.

HERBS

- Chamomile and Dandelion Root aid the digestive system. Liquorice can be added in small amounts where there is constipation, or to support the adrenal glands.
- Elderflowers and Eyebright will help to alleviate sneezing, itchy eyes and a runny nose.

- Nettles combined with Chamomile and Dandelion Root can be drunk freely for skin reactions and applied externally as a wash or compress.

ANAEMIA

Whatever the cause, anaemia results in the blood being less able to supply oxygen to the tissues. Symptoms include tiredness, lethargy and lack of colour. In children it is usually discovered when investigating frequent infections and poor weight gain.

Childhood anaemia is usually due to dietary iron deficiency. There is often folic acid and vitamin B12 deficiency as well.

Children require good iron reserves while they are developing, particularly during growth spurts and approaching puberty.

WHEN TO SEEK PROFESSIONAL HELP

- It is important to have a blood test to measure the haemoglobin levels and to rule out any serious underlying problems

DIET AND SUPPLEMENTS

- Processed convenience food and junk food high in sugar and salt rob the body of essential nutrients and should be strictly limited. All caffeine-containing drinks – tea, cola, chocolate – will inhibit the absorption of iron, especially when consumed with a meal. Bran and legumes (peas, beans and pulses) also inhibit iron absorption. It is for this reason that it is not a good idea to feed young children too many wholegrains in their diet.

- It is likely that any food intolerance (eg cow's milk or wheat) will affect the ability of the gut to absorb the necessary nutrients.

- Include unsulphured apricots, beetroot, black cherries and green leafy vegetables (especially raw) in the diet.

- Vitamin C improves the absorption of iron. It is interesting to note that fruit and vegetables high in iron also contain Vitamin C.

Free-range eggs are a well-balanced protein food and contain iron, vitamin B12 and folic acid. A traditional source of iron is liver, but this should be sourced from organically raised animals. Brewer's yeast, molasses and spirulina are good nutritional sources of iron and B vitamins. Floradix is an excellent supplement providing iron, B vitamins and vitamin C. Iron tablets can cause constipation or diarrhoea, natural sources are much easier for the body to assimilate.

HERBS

- Nettles, Dandelion Leaf and Raspberry Leaf provide iron.
- Angelica, Chamomile and Dandelion Root can be used to improve digestive function and absorption.

ANXIETY, nervousness, phobias

Alongside the obvious reasons for anxiety like starting or changing schools, exams and family problems, children can become anxious for various reasons. The true cause is often not obvious and anxiety can be masked by changes in behaviour, eg becoming difficult or withdrawn. Children don't find it easy to express their feelings and it is usually up to parents (and teachers) to pick up on the subtle signs, which is usually easier said than done.

Some children are born with a more nervous disposition than others. It is also challenging for children as they go through the various changes in their development, physically, mentally and emotionally and discovering what is expected of them. Growing up can be down right scary to those who don't like change or the face of a new challenge.

With young children films and television can have a very powerful effect on their psyche, the reason children like watching and listening to the same things over and over again is because it makes them feel secure and in control of the situation.

Herbs can help the transition through a difficult phase.

WHEN TO SEEK PROFESSIONAL HELP

- It is often helpful to seek the advice of a sympathetic practitioner who can give you an objective view.
- If the situation is not improving.

EXERCISE

- Fresh air and exercise can be a great antidote to anxiety.
- Simple breathing and relaxation techniques, yoga, martial arts, music and massage.

DIET AND SUPPLEMENTS

- Make sure the diet is wholesome and keep junk/processed foods to a minimum.
- Cut out caffeine-containing drinks – tea, chocolate and cola drinks which stimulate the nervous system.
- Avoid sugar and artificial sweeteners, additives and food colourings and rule out any food intolerances.
- A good children's multivitamin and mineral will help with any depletion or supplement a poor eater. Stress and anxiety depletes the body of essential nutrients.
- Include enough cold-pressed oil in the diet to support the nervous system.

HERBS

- Chamomile, Limeflowers and Lemon Balm help soothe and relax.
- Oats, Skullcap and Vervain are tonics to the nervous system.
- Stronger herbs like Valerian and Passionflower can be used when anxiety is marked.
- Essential oils of Chamomile, Lavender, Geranium and Rose can be used in a massage blend or in the bath.

ASTHMA

Asthma is a sudden and acute attack of breathlessness, caused by spasmodic constriction of the airways. It is characterised by a wheezy chest and difficulty with breathing out. In children it frequently presents itself with bouts of coughing at night. The accumulation of mucus in the airways as a result of inflammation or infection compounds the problem.

The cause is multifactorial with allergic, hereditary and emotional factors all playing a part. Viral and bacterial infections cause a significant proportion of asthma attacks. House dust and mites, feathers in pillows and duvets, animals, smoke, household sprays and cleaning fluids, perfumes, exhaust fumes, moulds, grasses and pollen, can all trigger an attack. The long-term use of steroids and inhalers can exacerbate the problem and affect the growth of a developing child. See also *Allergies* and *Coughs*.

WHEN TO SEEK PROFESSIONAL HELP

- Asthma is a potentially serious condition, and is best dealt with in conjuction with a practitioner, especially if the asthma is being controlled by orthodox drugs, and you wish to reduce any of these.

EXERCISE

- Deep breathing exercises are beneficial, playing a wind instrument can help.
- Gentle exercise, like walking and swimming help to improve lung capacity.
- Massage will help relieve tension and anxiety.

DIET AND SUPPLEMENTS

- Dairy products are the commonest cause of sensitivity and create a lot of mucus.
- Eggs, bananas, oranges, wheat and peanuts can also cause sensitivity.
- Avoid food additives and colourings like tartrazine (E102) and sulphur dioxide (E220).

HERBS

- Thyme is antispasmodic, antiseptic and an expectorant, so helps to dilate the airways and deal with mucus and any infection.

- Hyssop is a relaxing expectorant and antispasmodic.
- Cramp Bark and Valerian are antispasmodic and will help to relax the airways.
- Nebuliser oil (see page 40) can be used effectively to relieve congestion where the asthma is related to a chest infection.
- Caution: where the asthma is of a very allergic nature, proceed cautiously with the use of essential oils.

BEDWETTING

A child of four or five who is wetting the bed is most likely to be feeling insecure or unhappy about something. This might be due to starting school, a new baby in the family or moving house. It can also be due to an allergy to a food or environmental factor, or immature bladder control. Be comforting rather than scolding and don't make a fuss over a wet bed as this will only cause further upset.

WHEN TO SEEK PROFESSIONAL HELP

- If your child is still wetting the bed after the age of four it is advisable to check there is no structural abnormality of the urinary tract, or any underlying infection. A back problem could also be a factor. If the problem does not respond to the dietary and herbal advice seek further investigation into a food allergy, chemical sensitivity, e.g. chlorine in drinking water, or mineral deficiency.

DIET

- Avoid refined foods, sugar, caffeine-containing drinks like cola and additives that can cause bladder irritation and hence lack of control at night.

HERBS

- To soothe the bladder give Horsetail and Corn Silk
- St John's Wort can help the nervous control of the bladder.
- If the problem is linked with anxiety include Chamomile, Limeflowers or Lemon Balm in the mixture.
- Massage the lower back and abdomen with St John's Wort oil at bedtime. Chamomile or Lavender essential oil can be added to this.

CANDIDA / CANDIDIASIS

This is affecting more and more children. It is mostly attributable to the frequent use of antibiotics. Antibiotics, particularly the wide spectrum antibiotics which are used in young children, disrupt the beneficial bacteria in the gut.

A weakened immune system leaves the child susceptible to the over-growth of the yeast-like fungus Candida albicans which can cause inflammation in the gut, making the lining of the gut more permeable (leaky gut) and thereby allowing allergenic substances into the bloodstream. Toxins from the gut can also be absorbed through the gut into the body.

Candida can develop in the mouth or vagina. See also *Allergies* and *Thrush*.

WHEN TO SEEK PROFESSIONAL HELP

- It is important to establish whether or not candida is the problem, particularly before embarking on a very restricted diet.

DIET AND SUPPLEMENTS

- Sugar in every form should be avoided.
- Yeast-containing foods include bread, cheese, marmite, mushrooms and fermented foods like soya sauce. There is also yeast on the skins of fresh and dried fruit.
- Avoid supplements containing yeast, and meat that has been intensively reared using antibiotics, steroids and hormones.
- Eat plenty of fresh vegetables, including onions and garlic for their antifungal properties.
- Cold-pressed olive oil is anti-fungal.
- Include fresh pineapple, live plain yoghurt and/or Acidophilus in the diet.
- A restricted diet needs careful monitoring to avoid dietary deficiencies.

HERBS

- Angelica and Dandelion Root aid the digestive system.
- Echinacea, Golden Seal (buy from sustainable sources) and Marigold address the overgrowth of yeast as well as stimulating the immune system and lymphatics.

- Marjoram, Oregano, Rosemary and Thyme are antifungal and antioxidant.

CATARRH and SINUSITIS

The frontal sinuses are not fully developed in early childhood and sinusitis is rarely a cause of headache in the ten and unders. However, viral infections can lead to secondary bacterial infection and the nasal and maxillary sinuses may become filled with pus. Post-nasal drip and a recurrent chronic cough are the result of a chronic or recurrent infection.

Mucus is necessary to protect the lining of the mucous membranes from the environment. However, production can become excessive and it is then associated with irritated or inflamed mucous membranes. The cause can be related to the respiratory system, perhaps because of a cold or cough, or it may be related to diet. It usually signifies general congestion and overload in the body, often due to a digestive weakness. See also *Colds* and *Coughs*.

WHEN TO SEEK PROFESSIONAL HELP

- If the situation is chronic and does not respond to treatment.

DIET AND SUPPLEMENTS

- Avoid milk products, especially milk, cream and ice cream which will increase the amount of mucus the body is producing. Cow's milk, wheat, excess carbohydrate, refined carbohydrates and sugar can all be implicated in chronic problems.

HERBS

- Eyebright, Elderflowers and Ribwort Plantain help to tone the mucous membranes and deal with the catarrh.
- Use Echinacea and Golden Seal (buy from sustainable sources) to deal with infection.
- Elderflower, Peppermint and Composition Essence is invaluable where the mucus is entrenched.
- Spearmint is digestive and aids decongestion.
- Use Angelica and Dandelion Root to promote good digestion.

34

CHICKENPOX

This is a contagious viral illness which spreads via droplet infection (talking, coughing, sneezing) and through contact with pustular spots. It chiefly affects children under ten.

Chickenpox acquired by a mother who has not had it previously and contracts it during the eighth to fifteenth week of pregnancy or just before or after the birth can severely affect the baby.

The incubation period is 14–21 days and it is most contagious just before the spots appear until all the blisters have dried up.

First symptoms include headache, fever and malaise. The lymph glands might be swollen. The spots appear on the trunk first, then the face and limbs. The scalp, the inside of the mouth and throat, ears, soles of the feet and anus or vagina can be affected.

The spots turn into oval-shaped, fluid-filled blisters within 24 hours and dry up in a few days. These can be very itchy and every effort should be made to encourage your child not to scratch them, to prevent scarring and setting up any skin infection. The spots come in crops every 3–4 days so there are spots present in different stages at the same time. All the spots should dry up and the scabs fall off in 10 days. See also *Fever*.

WHEN TO SEEK PROFESSIONAL HELP

- If spots develop on the eyeball.
- If your child is on steroids or immunocompromised in any way.
- If your child feels unwell or there is vomiting, headache or malaise after the spots have healed.

DIET AND SUPPLEMENTS

- See *Diet during infections* on page 19.

HERBS

- Dab the spots with distilled Witch Hazel (which can be chilled) to alleviate the itching and help prevent infection.
- Golden Seal (buy from sustainable sources), Marigold and Myrrh tinctures make an effective lotion.
- Chamomile, Lavender, Peppermint and Tea Tree can be applied externally as an aromatic water, tea, tincture or essential oil. NB Use of Peppermint essential oil is best restricted for children under 2½ years old.

- Give Echinacea regularly during the acute stage.
- Cleavers and Marigold can be given internally during the eruptive period.
- A healing cream of St John's Wort oil, comfrey, marigold and lavender essential oil is ideal to counter scarring.

CHRONIC FATIGUE SYNDROME

This is becoming more prevalent among children and adolescents. It usually follows a viral illness which reduces cell respiration. This affects the muscles and the legs feel achy and tire easily, making walking an effort. There is general fatigue and adequate rest and sleep are required. Over exertion will lead to poor concentration and brain fog.

It is essential to investigate why the virus has been able to become established. Glandular fever is a common culprit, but any viral illness or a chronic recurrent condition like tonsillitis can be a factor in the depletion leading to CFS. Other factors include environmental pollutants, stress and vaccinations. Treatment needs to address diet and the digestive system and the immune system. See also *Glandular fever, Candida/Candidiasis.*

WHEN TO SEEK PROFESSIONAL HELP

- This is best approached with a qualified practitioner.

DIET AND SUPPLEMENTS

- Beetroot improves cell respiration, mix with apple or grape juice.
- Coenzyme Q10 is a supplement that improves cell respiration.
- Essential fatty acids are important, include cold-pressed oils like linseed and olive in the diet.

HERBS

- Angelica, Chinese Angelica, Ginseng and Vervain are important tonic herbs.
- Marjoram, Oregano, Rosemary and Thyme are anti-oxidant herbs.

COLDS

Babies and young children tend to get regular colds, it is part of developing their immune systems which are immature.

Repeated colds tend to strike when resistance is at its lowest. They are most common in winter when children don't spend so much time outdoors in the fresh air and tend to be cooped up in centrally heated houses or stuffy classrooms. See also *Catarrh and Sinusitis, Coughs* and *Fever*.

DIET AND SUPPLEMENTS

- See *Diet during infections* on page 19.
- A Children's multivitamin and mineral or Vitamin C with rosehips over the winter months can be helpful.

HERBS

- Echinacea and Olive Leaf boost the immune system.
- Elderflowers are good to give as a tea to alleviate congestion.
- Elderberry and Rosehips are rich in Vitamin C and excellent as a winter booster.

COLIC

Many babies suffer from colic, most commonly in the first three months of life when the digestive system is adapting to life outside the womb. It is usually worst in the evening, when all concerned are tired.

Colic can be due to the baby not being correctly latched onto the nipple or feeding too quickly, so swallowing a lot of air with the milk.

With bottlefed babies it can be due to an allergy to the formula milk or air from the bottle. Feeding too frequently can exacerbate the problem.

WHEN TO SEEK PROFESSIONAL HELP

- Seek advice from your midwife or a breast-feeding counsellor.

- Cranial osteopathy can dramatically help colic and improve latching on. It will alleviate any residual pressure caused by the forces exerted during the birth process, particularly on the head and neck.

- An Acupuncturist can show you how to moxa and warm your baby's tummy to alleviate colic.

DIET AND SUPPLEMENTS

- If you are breast-feeding avoiding the foods you went off during pregnancy, or those you know you have sensitivities to (like cow's milk) can help.

- Onions, garlic, beans, lentils, cabbage and spicy foods often upset a baby's tummy.

- Make sure you don't compromise your diet by cutting too many things out while breast-feeding.

- Place one teaspoon of bicarbonate of soda in a glass of cooled, boiled water, stir until completely dissolved and give one to two teaspoons as required to break up the wind.

HERBS

- Fennel and Dill Seed (the components of gripe water) are carminitive which means they reduce intestinal wind.

- Chamomile, Lemon Balm and Limeflowers are relaxing herbs.

- Angelica can help improve digestive function, it is warming and carminitive.

- All the above can be drunk liberally as teas by mum if solely breast-feeding or given to baby a teaspoon at a time.

- Use Chamomile and Lavender essential oils diluted to massage baby's tummy.

CONJUCTIVITIS

This is inflammation of the protective membrane of the eye, caused by an infection, an allergy or a foreign body in the eye. Typically, this is associated with a cold in small children, where they have a runny nose and wipe their face then rub their eyes. The whites of the eye become pink or red, are sore and irritate. The eyelids can become puffy. Where there is an infection, they can become weepy, with the eyelids sticking together after sleep. Care must be taken not to spread any infection to the other eye or other members of the family.

WHEN TO SEEK PROFESSIONAL HELP

- Make sure of the diagnosis and commence treatment rapidly. Eyes are delicate organs and the situation can deteriorate rapidly.

HERBS

- A sore inflamed eye can be soothed with an eyewash using equal parts of Eyebright and Marigold. Chamomile might also be used. For any infection Marigold needs to be included in the mix. If making up an infusion simmer the herbs for a few minutes in a saucepan to sterilize.
- Alternatively dilute 1 part distilled Witch Hazel in 3 to 5 parts boiled water and use as an eyebath.
- A few grains of sea salt can be added to each eyebathful. If using an eyebath use a clean eyebath and fresh solution for each eye. Otherwise, use a fresh piece of cotton wool for each eye and swab with the solution. This should be done 2-4 times a day.
- A fresh mixture should be made up each day.

CONSTIPATION

It is common for babies to become constipated when solids are introduced into their diet. It takes time to adjust to a non liquid diet and different foods which might not all suit. Make sure they get plenty of fluids – either milk (breast or formula), herb teas or water. Pureed fruit like apple, apricots, dates and prunes can help.

In older children, tension can be a major factor, perhaps not having enough time before school, or an emotional upset.

Bottlefed babies might have difficulty digesting or an intolerance to their formula milk causing constipation.

Babies who are solely breast-fed might only have one bowel movement a week but they are not considered constipated, although things might get uncomfortable in the build up to an evacuation. See also *Colic*.

HERBS

● Angelica aids digestion.

● Chamomile tea is a gentle and relaxing digestive.

● Dandelion Root and Liquorice are gentle laxatives suitable for children.

COUGHS

A cough frequently accompanies an infection, but can be due to excess mucus, nervousness or an irritant. See also *Catarrh* and *Colds*.

WHEN TO SEEK PROFESSIONAL HELP

● If the cough persists for more than two weeks, if there are any difficulties with breathing, or if your child is coughing up mucus, especially if coloured yellow, green or streaked with blood.

HERBS

● Hyssop, Ribwort Plantain and Coltsfoot are helpful where the child has a tendency to get a lot of coughs.

● Eucalyptus and Thyme are important antiseptics.

● Liquorice and Marshmallow are soothing.

● Essential oils of Eucalyptus smithii, Thymus saturoides and Tea Tree are gentle enough to use in a nebuliser or oil burner and rub onto the chest. I use a blend of these three to make what I call the Nebuliser oil.

CRADLECAP

This is a yellow scaly condition of the scalp caused by the over production of sebum that is common in babies. It can be crusty, or feel quite oily.

Olive oil, if nothing else is on hand, can be massaged into the scalp to help gently lift off the scales. Picking at it dry can lead to bleeding and infection and generally makes it worse.

With little interference it will usually diminish, but sometimes it will spread and it can be a precursor to eczema and psoriasis in the future.

HERBS

- Chamomile, Lavender and Rosemary essential oils in a base of Chamomile, Marigold or Almond oil makes a gentle oil to massage into the scalp. This will loosen the scales which can then be washed out with a mild herbal baby shampoo like Chamomile or Marigold.

- Cleavers, Nettles and Heartsease are gentle cleansers which can be given as teas internally, as well as used to wash the scalp, if the cradlecap is extensive.

CROUP

Ostensibly a viral infection, commonly caused by the flu virus. The larynx, trachea and bronchi are all involved in the inflammatory process. Symptoms start with a mild fever and runny nose. In the older child the symptoms progress to a sore throat, difficulty with swallowing and a dry, irritating cough. The younger child has a relatively small airway and the resultant swelling and secretions can severely obstruct breathing. It is characterised by a barking cough and a respiratory noise, particularly on inspiration (croup) which usually starts in the middle of the night. The natural tendency for the airway to collapse on breathing in is increased by the child's desperate attempts to overcome the obstruction, thus exacerbating the situation. Parental anxiety exacerbates the situation further.

Some children get recurrent bouts of croup for a number of years, usually whenever they have a cold. These children have particularly floppy airways.

Croup can seem akin to asthma, but asthma drugs are no help. Antibiotics are of no help either.

A warm confident environment and plenty of reassurance for the child is important. Keep the air moist. See also *Coughs* and *Colds*.

WHEN TO SEEK PROFESSIONAL HELP

- For reassurance as this situation can be extremely scary for all involved.
- If the child is breathing rapidly and the lips or face are blue.

HERBS

- Thyme will help to deal with the infection and relax the airways.
- Give relaxing teas of Chamomile, Lavender, Lemon Balm and Limeflowers.
- Cramp Bark and Valerian are antispasmodics which will relax the airways.
- Use Chamomile and Lavender essential oils in a warm bath or steam bath to relax.
- Thyme, Eucalyptus and Tea Tree essential oils, see Nebuliser oil on page 40, can be employed to good effect and added to a steam bath.
- Bach Flower Rescue Remedy can be taken by the child or parent for fear and anxiety.
- If your child is prone to croup treat a cold or cough as soon as it manifests.

CYSTITIS

Urinary tract infections are more common in girls than boys. Structural abnormalities are not uncommon but are usually picked up on prenatal scans or shortly after birth. They are most frequently caused by bacteria from the bowel, often aided by wiping from back to front rather than front to back. Vaginal infections like thrush can also predispose to cystitis.

Symptoms include frequent urination, urgency to get to the toilet and burning pain on passing water which reduces young children to tears. Bed-wetting and strong smelling and cloudy urine indicate a problem.

WHEN TO SEEK PROFESSIONAL HELP

- It is imperative to treat the infection promptly as it can spread up the tubules to the kidneys.
- Low back pain or tummy pain, headache or fever indicate a kidney infection.
- If the symptoms do not improve in a couple of days.
- If blood is being passed.

DIET AND SUPPLEMENTS

- It is important to drink plenty throughout the day. Water, sugar-free cranberry juice and barley water. Barley water can be made by simmering 50g (2oz) of barley in 500ml (1 pint) of water until soft. Add honey and lemon to taste. ½ tsp of bicarbonate of soda in a glass of water will help to alkalize acidic urine.
- Avoid sugar and sugary foods.

HERBS

- Corn Silk and Marshmallow Leaf will help to soothe cystitis. Couchgrass is soothing and anti-microbial.
- Buchu and Bearberry (Uva-ursi) are specific antiseptics for the urinary system. Echinacea could be used if it is the only thing available.
- Horsetail helps to strengthen the bladder and urinary tract and can be useful if cystitis is a recurrent problem.
- Parsley Piert and Pellitory-of-the-Wall have a restorative effect on the kidneys and can help protect the kidneys during infection. It is important to include one of these herbs if there is a history of kidney disease or underlying structural abnormalities of the urinary tract.

DIARRHOEA

This is the body's attempt to expel an irritant from the bowel, commonly caused by an infection, food poisoning or parasites. Antibiotics, especially broad-spectrum ones, can cause diarrhoea by upsetting the balance of the gut flora. A bout of diarrhoea in itself will upset the gut flora and can prolong the diarrhoea.

Recurrent diarrhoea can be a sign of a food intolerance, usually cow's milk or wheat, or poor fat digestion and will need further investigation.

WHEN TO SEEK PROFESSIONAL HELP

- Babies and young children need special attention as they easily become dehydrated – signs such as lethargy, sunken eyes, a depressed fontanelle in babies and loss of skin elasticity need urgent treatment.
- If the diarrhoea is particularly violent, and accompanied by pain, vomiting, a high temperature or blood loss.
- If it does not improve within 24 to 36 hours.
- If it is recurrent.

DIET AND SUPPLEMENTS

- Maintaining fluid levels is vital. Infants are particularly susceptible to dehydration as they have a higher percentage of body water, a higher metabolic rate and a larger surface area to volume.
- Dioralyte, which can be obtained from a chemist, will replace lost fluids and salts. Alternatively make up a drink using one part apple, grape or orange juice diluted with three parts water, with a pinch of salt added to it.
- Live yoghurt or Acidophilus powder will help to re-establish the gut flora and normal bowel movements.
- It is best to limit the diet to fluids until the worst is over.

HERBS

- Chamomile helps to soothe and settle the digestive system, this can be mixed with Spearmint.
- Barberry (Berberis) is excellent for gut infections, but is bitter to taste so just a few drops in disguise, or as capsules in older children.

- Echinacea and Garlic are also effective anti-microbial agents.
- Meadowsweet is soothing and anti-inflammatory.
- Slippery Elm as powder or tablets helps to absorb toxins and soothe a sore gut.

EARACHE/EAR INFECTIONS

Earache commonly becomes apparent in babies and young children with ear rubbing or pulling. As the situation becomes more acute the child can become quite distressed with crying and screaming, or they are just obviously out of sorts. Children might become noticeably deaf.

Pain in and around the ear is caused by infection or inflammation occurring in the middle ear. It can also be due to referred pain from the teeth. Babies and young children are particularly prone to ear infections, as their relatively short eustachian tubes easily become blocked if there is a catarrhal infection, or if the tonsils or glands are swollen.

Apart from the distress of seeing a child in pain there is a risk of infection spreading to the bony parts of the ear, so treatment needs to be prompt. If the ear drum perforates the discharge is usually watery or mucousy. This relieves the pressure and hence the pain.

Antibiotics may appear to resolve the situation quickly but they are not the answer for recurrent ear infections. They tend to drive the infection deeper and don't address the underlying problem. Trials have shown that they have no positive effect on the resolution of the condition and that they can compound the situation leading to glue ear. See also *Catarrh and Sinusitis, Colds, Coughs* and *Glue ear.*

WHEN TO SEEK PROFESSIONAL HELP
- It is best to have any suspected ear infection checked out.
- If there is bleeding or discharge from the ear.
- If the problem is recurrent.

DIET
- If the condition is recurrent it is quite likely to be associated with a food intolerance eg cow's milk.

HERBS

- Mullein, St John's Wort or Garlic oil, preferably warmed, make excellent eardrops. Put 2 drops in each ear (even if only one ear is hurting). Lavender essential oil might be added to any of the above. Use 1 drop of essential oil per 1ml of base oil for added effect.

- If the eardrum is perforated do not use eardrops, clean the ear of any discharge and put a drop or two of Lavender essential oil on a piece of cotton wool and place that in the ear.

- Inhalation of essential oils like Eucalyptus, Tea Tree and Thyme, which are antiseptic is useful.

- Pasque Flower (Pulsatilla) or Homoeopathic Pulsatilla given orally can help alleviate the pain.

- Elderflower, Peppermint and Composition Essence can help break up the congestion in the ear. It is very hot to taste but can be useful in small amounts with other herbs in young children.

- To ease the pain heat a cup of salt and place in a cloth. When just cool enough hold the pack over the ear until cool.

- Echinacea and Golden Seal (buy from sustainable sources) should be taken every 1-3 hours while the condition is acute.

ECZEMA

This is irritation and inflammation of the skin. Causes might be external, like irritants in washing powders, but hereditary, dietary and emotional factors can all play their part. Treatment involves assessing all the factors, and internal remedies including diet are vital alongside external remedies to soothe the skin. See also *Allergies*.

WHEN TO SEEK PROFESSIONAL HELP

- Treatment is best undertaken with a qualified Herbalist, especially when steroid creams are being used. Eczema can become seriously infected.

DIET AND SUPPLEMENTS

- Any food intolerances, eg cow's milk, need to be identified and addressed.

- Cold-pressed oils need to be included in the diet to supply the essential fatty acids vital for the health of the skin. Borage (Starflower), Evening Primrose and Hemp Seed oil are particularly good for the skin.

HERBS

- Borage (Starflower) or Hemp seed oil cream is usually the most effective for soothing dry, irritated skin.
- Chamomile as a compress or cream can help when the skin is very inflamed.
- Marigold (Calendula) cream is useful where there is a risk of infection or to help heal broken areas.
- Floral waters of Chamomile, Yarrow and Tea Tree can be sprayed onto the skin. This is particularly useful where the eczema is wet and weeping and there is a risk of infection. Using a plant sprayer or atomiser avoids further distress to sore areas.
- Distilled Witch Hazel is soothing and cooling.
- An Oat bath can be used to soothe inflamed skin, especially if the eczema is extensive. Put 150g (6oz) of porridge oats into a cotton or muslin bag or handkerchief and tie underneath the hot water tap. Squeeze the soaked bag to release the milky emollient liquid.
- Nettles are particularly helpful where there is a strong allergic element. They are also a blood cleanser and nutritive.
- Cleavers is also a cleanser, specifically for the lymphatic system.
- Angelica and Dandelion Root aid digestive function which is often implicated in eczema.

FEVER

Fever is Nature's way of helping the body fight off infection and shouldn't be suppressed unnecessarily; however, the fever needs to be monitored carefully. Babies and young children haven't got a fully developed temperature control mechanism, and some children are particularly prone to febrile convulsions with any temperature change up until the age of six. In such cases the temperature shouldn't be allowed to go above 39°C (102°F).

Keep your child as comfortable as possible, taking clothes off when too hot and covering with just a sheet. The room should be kept neither too hot or too cold. Use cool compresses of teas made with the herbs given below on your child's forehead and feet. If the temperature goes above 39°C (102°F) bathe your child with tepid water (cold water actually reduces the body's ability to lose heat by closing the pores) and sponging with the same herbs. Some of the infectious diseases will cause a fever that peaks at 40-40.5°C (104-105°F).

Treat any accompanying symptoms and infection accordingly, eg *Colds* and *Coughs*.

WHEN TO SEEK PROFESSIONAL HELP

- If your child suffers a convulsion.
- If the fever is intermittent.
- If your child is suffering from repeated fevers.
- A child who has had a febrile convulsion shouldn't receive the whooping cough vaccine.

DIET AND SUPPLEMENTS

- Plenty of fluids are necessary to prevent dehydration, give sips of liquid frequently.

HERBS

- Elderflowers, Limeflowers and Yarrow help to lower a fever by promoting sweating.
- Catmint is cooling and will help to reduce a fever, give hourly.
- Spearmint is also cooling.

FLU

See *Colds, Coughs, Fevers, Headaches* and *Sore throat*.

GASTROENTERITIS

See *Diarrhoea*.

GERMAN MEASLES – Rubella

Spread by droplet infection, the incubation period is 2 to 3 weeks. Although mild in children, it tends to affect older children, adolescents and young adults more severely. If it develops during the first four months of pregnancy, it can cause congenital malformation, such as heart or mental defects, deafness or cataracts.

There might be a runny nose, sore throat and slight fever, but the disease is not usually suspected until the rash appears as small, flat pink spots behind the ears and on the forehead. It then spreads rapidly to the trunk and then to the limbs.

If the rash is dense the skin looks red and it may be itchy for a few days. Tender enlargement of the glands in the neck and behind the ears usually occurs. Mild conjuctivitis is common.

The illness lasts 2 to 3 days at most, and can pass virtually unnoticed, making treatment unneccessary. Complications are rare, transient arthritis may occur in adolescents.

DIET AND SUPPLEMENTS

- See *Diet during infections* on page 19.

HERBS

- Give Burdock, Cleavers, Marigold and Echinacea to aid the immune system.
- Distilled Witch Hazel or aromatic waters of Chamomile or Lavender can be used on the skin to alleviate any itching.

GLANDULAR FEVER

This virus usually strikes during the teenage years, around exams or other stressful times, but it can occur in children too. The incubation period is 7–10 days plus and it is mildly infectious. The virus affects the lymphatic system.

Flu-like symptoms occur during the first part of the illness, followed by debility, inability to concentrate and depression. Tiredness, malaise, headache, intermittent fever and sweating, swollen glands in the neck and sometimes abdomen, sore throat (with red spots) and a rash in the first 10 days are all early symptoms. Hepatitis, enlarged spleen and viral meningitis are not uncommon.

A blood test will confirm the diagnosis but may not prove positive if taken in the post viral phase when the virus is no longer active. The virus can reoccur and remain latent in the immunocompromised.

It is a prolonged illness and the convalescent period shouldn't be rushed. Slowly build up the amount of excercise that is done and do not push things as it can turn the tiredness into a chronic state which causes longterm debility. See also *Fever, Chronic Fatigue Syndrome* and *Tonsillitis*.

WHEN TO SEEK PROFESSIONAL HELP

● It is wise to have help from the beginning in order to lessen the extent of the illness and prevent the possibility of post viral chronic fatigue syndrome.

DIET AND SUPPLEMENTS

● Organic beetroot as juice, raw or cooked root.

● Floradix, Spirulina and Vitamin C are beneficial supplements.

● See *Diet during infections* on page 19.

HERBS

● Echinacea and Wild Indigo for the immune system.

● Cleavers and Marigold for the lymphatic system.

● Boneset for the fever.

● Dandelion Root and Milk Thistle for the liver and digestive system.

● Liquorice for constipation and to support the adrenal glands.

● Use essential oils of Eucalyptus, Lavender, Pine, Rosemary and Thyme in the bath and oil burners during the acute period.

● Ginseng (not during the acute phase), Nettles, Oats and Vervain for convalescence.

GLUE EAR

Glue ear occurs after recurrent ear infections. Antibiotics don't completely resolve the infection each time and there is a gradual build up of exudate in the middle ear. This chronic congestion leads to hearing loss which develops slowly with the child seemingly becoming inattentive, particularly at school. The orthodox treatment is grommets.

Treatment of glue ear has to be sustained over a number of months to be effective and needs to involve dietary changes. Passive smoking and polluted environments contribute towards the incidence of glue ear. See also *Earache, Catarrh and Sinusitis*.

WHEN TO SEEK PROFESSIONAL HELP

- Since there is no quick fix it is best to see a practitioner to make sure you are on the right track and to monitor the situation.

DIET AND SUPPLEMENTS

- Food intolerances need to be investigated – cow's milk, wheat, tomatoes (ketchup). Mucus-forming foods like milk products, sugar, refined carbohydrates, oranges, peanuts need to be kept to a minimum.
- Try to include garlic and onions in the daily diet. Lemon and apple cider vinegar can help to clear the mucus.
- Make sure there is no constipation.

EXERCISE

- Plenty of fresh air and enough exercise help to stimulate the circulation and lymphatic system and boost the immune system. Massage of the head and neck around the ear helps to stimulate the blood and lymphatics and aid decongestion.

HERBS

- Echinacea and Golden Seal address the infection and boost the immune system. Golden Seal (buy from sustainable sources) tones the mucous membranes.
- Elderflower, Peppermint and Composition Essence is essential, even in small doses.
- Essential oils of Eucalyptus, Tea tree, Chamomile and Lavender can be used in a massage oil or in an inhalation. See Nebuliser oil on page 40.

HEADACHE, Migraine

These tend to manifest as children get older and occur more frequently with infections as the frontal sinuses develop. Girls become more prone to headaches around puberty.

Migraine usually begins as a digestive disturbance in younger children who develop the headaches and visual disturbance as they get older. If headaches are recurrent there is likely to be a digestive weakness or some stress causing anxiety. See also *Allergies, Anxiety* and *Catarrh and Sinusitis*.

WHEN TO SEEK PROFESSIONAL HELP

● If the headache comes after an accident or blow to the head.

● If associated with photophobia and/or a stiff neck.

● To rule out any structural misalignment with the neck or back.

DIET

● Cut out caffeine containing food and drinks like chocolate, cola, coffee and tea which can cause headaches.

● Limit fast food, sugary foods and fizzy drinks. Avoid food colourings, additives and artificial sweeteners.

● Rule out any food intolerances like cow's milk or wheat.

● Cheese and oranges can be a trigger.

● Make sure children drink plenty of fluids, preferably as water or diluted pure juices as dehydration will cause headaches.

HERBS

● Californian Poppy, Lavender and Passionflower are relaxing herbs to alleviate the pain.

● Skullcap and Wood Betony are tonic and restorative to the nervous system.

● Angelica and Dandelion Root will aid digestive function.

● Lavender essential oil can be rubbed into the temples, neat.

HEAD LICE

Headlice come in plagues and are indiscriminate about who they live on. They move via close contact and spread easily via long hair, sharing hats and brushes etc. They can live for 24 hours away from the body. The louse is a pale greyish brown while the eggs (the nits) are visible as white specks glued to the hair shaft close to the scalp. The eggs hatch after eight days and each louse lives up to 5 weeks. Headlice can become endemic among some school children and can seem immune to treatment.

Keep hair brushes, hats, towels and pillows separate. Tie long hair back. Headlice can cause bites on the head and back of the neck which can become infected. Some children are particularly sensitive.

Put plenty of conditioner on your child's hair and comb through with a nit comb thoroughly at least once or twice a week during infestations, and preferably once a week as a preventative measure, especially when you know other children who have them.

HERBS

- Quassia has been shown in trials to kill headlice, it will not however kill the eggs (or nits), so the process has to be repeated until after the eggs have hatched. This can be applied in a shampoo and conditioner, as tincture added to shampoo or sprayed on, or as a final hair rinse made from simmering the chips of bark to make a decoction.

- Ideally use a coconut-based shampoo or Tea Tree or Quassia shampoo. A conditioner is important, preferably Tea Tree, Neem or Quassia. Use at least twice a week for a week and combine with conditioning and combing. Then repeat after one week and use as a precautionary measure weekly if there are headlice at school.

- Essential oils of Eucalyptus, Lavender, Tea Tree, Thyme and Rosemary can be used in a base oil such as olive oil at a dose of 1 drop of essential oil per 1ml of base oil. 20-50mls of oil (depending on the length and thickness of the hair) will be required to apply to all the hair. Wrap the head in cling film and wash out the next morning.

HICCUPS

This is usually caused by rushing food and drink which ferments in the stomach causing irritation and spasms of the diaphragm. Recurrent bouts suggest a digestive weakness and poor fat digestion. Drinking too much at mealtimes can aggravate the problem. Anxiety can be a factor, as can antibiotic treatment which disrupts the gut flora. Please see *Colic* for appropriate herbs.

HYPERACTIVITY

Having a child who is hyperactive is exhausting for parents and can cause misery and despair. A child who is overactive, restless, easily excitable, lacks concentration and seems to need little sleep is likely to be hyperactive. Their behaviour can become aggressive or disruptive. Diagnosis can be difficult with varying degrees of hyperactivity. A demanding child who gets bored easily might simply be highly intelligent.

The most common cause of hyperactivity is food related and there is frequently a family history of allergies. Environmental toxins can be a factor, particularly a build up of heavy metals in the system (see page 55). The problems can go back to exposure to chemicals while in the womb, or difficulties with the birth. Poor digestion with either loose stools or constipation can be an indication of a food intolerance or toxicity and will compound the problem. Overuse of antibiotics might have led to the overgrowth of candida. These factors irritate the nervous system and adversely affect brain function. The strategy to take is one of removing the irritants and soothe, calm and heal the nervous system. See also *Allergies, Candida/Candidiasis* and *Sleeplessness*.

WHEN TO SEEK PROFESSIONAL HELP

- Support is advisable if the hyperactivity is severe.
- If dietary recommendations and gentle herbs don't work.
- If making major dietary changes.

DIET

- Foods that generally compound the problem are sugar and artificial sweeteners, caffeine-containing food and drink like tea, chocolate and cola drinks, and food additives and colourings like tartrazine. Cow's milk products, wheat, eggs and oranges are frequently implicated.

- Food intolerances or an inadequate diet will lead to nutritional deficiencies and susceptibility to heavy metal toxicity. A good quality multivitamin and mineral specifically designed for hyperactive children will provide the necessary levels of all the elements. The B vitamins, magnesium and zinc are among the elements vital to healthy brain function.

- Include cold-pressed oils like olive and flax in the diet to provide the essential fatty acids vital to the function of the nervous system.

- Oats are beneficial to the nervous system and can be included in the diet as porridge and oat-based cereals.

HERBS

- Chamomile, Lemon balm and Limeflowers are all calming and soothing.

- Skullcap and Vervain are tonic to the nervous system.

- Lavender, Passionflower and Valerian are stronger herbs to be used only after trying those above.

- Use Angelica, Dandelion Root and Liquorice to promote the function of the digestive system.

- Essential oils of Chamomile and Lavender can be used in an oil burner in the room during the day or night, in the bath or in a massage oil.

IMPETIGO

This contagious skin infection is caused by the Staphylococcus bacteria and needs prompt anti-infective treatment. Early diagnosis and treatment is important to prevent the problem spreading. It typically affects the lips, chin and nose where it starts off as weeping blisters that form a characteristic golden-yellow crust. Touching them can quickly spread the infection to other parts of the body or other children.

DIET AND SUPPLEMENTS

- If the problem is recurrent there is probably a factor in the diet like sugar to address.

HERBS

- Golden Seal (buy from sustainable sources), Marigold and Myrrh externally.
- Give Echinacea and Wild Indigo internally.
- Essential oils of Tea Tree and Thyme can be applied neat, but can sting. Alternatively dilute in Garlic, Marigold, St John's Wort or any vegetable oil, use 5 drops of essential oil per ml of oil. Apply 2-4 times a day.

MEASLES

Measles is a highly contagious viral illness which is spread by droplet infection – talking, coughing and sneezing. The incubation period is 8-14 days and it is infectious from 7 days after infection to 10 days after the rash has started. It starts similarly to a cold with nasal catarrh, sneezing, red, watering eyes, swollen eyelids and a headache. A cough and hoarseness, due to laryngitis, and photophobia (sensitivity to light) come by the second day.

Koplik's spots, white spots surrounded by a red area of inflammation inside the cheeks are diagnostic of measles. During the third or fourth day of the highly infectious catarrhal stage, the rash starts behind the ears and hairline and rapidly appears over the rest of the body, accompanied by a high temperature which can reach 40°C (104°F). These flat, brownish-red spots fuse to form the characteristic blotchy rash which usually covers the face too. The rash does not generally itch. The rash is fully erupted in 2-3 days and the fever subsides as the rash disappears. Swollen lymph nodes in the neck, vomiting and diarrhoea, abdominal pain and earache can occur.

Among well nourished children most cases are uncomplicated, but middle ear infection and pneumonia can occur due to secondary infection, and persistent conjuctivitis can lead to corneal damage if neglected. Encephalitis is a rare complication. The child should feel better in 7-10 days. See also *Fever* and *Conjuctivitis*.

WHEN TO SEEK PROFESSIONAL HELP

• Measles is a notifiable disease, so contact your GP as well as your Herbalist.

• If the child isn't feeling better after a week.

• If the temperature starts to rise again.

DIET AND SUPPLEMENTS

• See *Diet during infections* on page 19.

• Give carrots, carrot juice and beetroot juice to boost the immune system and provide betacarotene. If necessary give a multivitamin containing betacarotene and Vitamin C. Betacarotene is a precursor to Vitamin A, and is a safer supplement for children as Vitamin A can be toxic at excessive levels.

• Vitamin A deficiency is linked to increased severity of the disease and eye problems.

HERBS

• Give Echinacea regularly during the acute stage.

• Burdock and Nettles help to encourage toxins out of the system.

• Cleavers and Marigold boost the lymphatic drainage.

• Use Eucalyptus and Lavender essential oils in the bath.

• Bathe eyes, if sore, with cold compresses of Elderflowers or Chamomile.

MOLLUSCUM

Molluscum contagiosum is a viral skin infection that produces wart-like spots on the skin. These can spread steadily and infect other susceptible members of the family and be stubbornly difficult to get rid of.

HERBS

- Internally Echinacea and Marigold to boost the immune system.
- Dandelion Root and Vervain are useful tonics if your child is rundown.
- Externally apply tincture or cream of Marigold, Propolis and Thuja.
- Essential oils of Myrrh and Tea Tree can be used externally.

MOUTH ULCERS

These often manifest at the end of an illness or when your child is a bit run down, perhaps after an illness or at the end of the school term.

DIET AND SUPPLEMENTS

- Make sure there are plenty of fresh fruit and vegetables in the diet. Vitamins C and B complex can become depleted during stressful times.

HERBS

- Echinacea for the immune system
- Dandelion Root and Vervain are helpful tonics.
- Marigold, Myrrh and Golden Seal (buy from sustainable sources) can be applied to the ulcers neat with a cotton bud to good effect. If the ulcers are large this might sting too much so dilute as necessary.

MUMPS

This viral illness, spread by droplet infection, usually affects school children and young adults. The incubation period is 18 days with a gradual onset of symptoms. Initial symptoms are chills, fever, malaise, headache, loss of appetite and aching muscles. Pain under the ears and jaw begins about 24 hours later, the salivary glands can become extremely sore and swollen after this.

Fever, malaise and spasms of the jaw muscles are followed by swelling of one or both of the parotid glands (palpable at the angle of the jaw) sometimes one after the other. Swelling of the glands can in fact be the first symptom. The submandibular glands (under the jaw) may also be swollen. Jaw movement may be extremely painful making eating and drinking difficult. Swelling lasts for about a week or less. Fever is moderate 38.3 to 38.9°C (101-102°F). The symptoms subside in a few days and may be followed by the swelling of a previously unaffected gland. See also *Fever*.

WHEN TO SEEK PROFESSIONAL HELP

• If abdominal or testicular pain occurs .

• If a severe headache or stiff neck develops.

DIET AND SUPPLEMENTS

• See *Diet during infections* on page 19.

• Give foods that are easy to swallow like juices and soup.

HERBS

• Give Cleavers and Marigold to aid the lymphatic tissue.

• Echinacea should be given every 2 to 3 hours.

• Californian Poppy, Cramp Bark and Passionflower can help ease the discomfort.

• Compresses of any of the above can be applied externally over the neck.

NAPPY RASH

Nappy rash is caused by the interaction of the urine and stool next to the skin. It can be made worse by some foods making the stool or urine stronger.

Disposable nappies contain gels and other chemicals that react with the urine and can cause nappy rash in sensitive children. When using cotton washable nappies use a non-biological washing powder (it is hard to remove all traces of the enzymes in biological powders), and avoid chlorine-based bleaching agents.

Children with allergies or skin conditions and cradlecap tend to be more prone to nappy rash and the rash is often worse during teething.

HERBS

- Protect the bottom from irritating substances by using an oil-based product, eg a Beeswax and Calendula oil ointment at night to create a protective layer, and allow air over the area during the day as much as possible.

- Wash the nappy area with a strong infusion of Marigold tea.

- St John's Wort oil with Lavender essential oil is healing and protective.

ROSEOLA

Usually an illness in the under twos. The child develops a high fever, often without appearing particularly ill. Due to the high temperature convulsions are not uncommon with roseola. There is mild swelling of the lymph glands. After three to four days the temperature suddenly drops and the rash appears which lasts no more than a day or two, followed by a rapid recovery. See *Fever* for treatment.

SLEEPLESSNESS

Children need to sleep at least 15 hours a day as new born, gradually reducing to about 8-10 hours as a 12 year old (with variation obviously), if they are not having anything like this then there must be something keeping them awake. Certain foods can irritate the system preventing restful sleep. Chemicals in the form of additives, colourings and preservatives, or chemicals in the environment can do the same.

With babies over 6 months old sleep training can work well to break the habit, but you will need to make allowances for teething and illness. For older children try to have a set bedtime routine with enough time to wind down, a relaxing bath, stories and perhaps a relaxing tape to listen to in bed. See also *Anxiety* and *Hyperactivity*.

WHEN TO SEEK PROFESSIONAL HELP

- If the situation is intractable seek help, sleep deprivation is unhealthy for you and your child.
- To rule out any underlying medical problem.

DIET AND SUPPLEMENTS

- Avoid caffeine-containing food and drink – chocolate, cola drinks, tea and coffee which easily overstimulate children. Cut out foods with additives and colourings and avoid sugary foods which make for excess energy.
- Investigate any food intolerances.

HERBS

- Chamomile can work beautifully. Use it as tea in a bottle or cup for babies and as normal tea for older children.
- Lavender, Lemon Balm and Limeflowers are relaxing and sleep inducing.
- Any of the above can be used as bath herbs.
- Use stronger herbs like Passionflower and Valerian in the short-term for older children if the ones above aren't helping, or for stressful times like exams where anxiety is disrupting sleep.
- Chamomile or Lavender essential oils can be used in the bath, a massage oil or in an oil burner in the bedroom.
- A Hop or Lavender pillow at night can be very effective.

SORE THROAT

Sore throats and difficulty in swallowing accompany many childhood infections and coughs and colds. Inflammation of the throat can involve the voice box, the larynx, causing hoarseness or loss of voice – laryngitis. Persistant sore throats usually suggest an irritant or allergy. See also *Colds, Coughs* and *Tonsillitis*.

HERBS

- Marshmallow and Liquorice can help to soothe the throat.
- Sage and Thyme can be used as a gargle if the child is old enough, otherwise sprays can be helpful.
- Propolis products are very effective.

TEETHING

Although teething can cause little trouble in some, for others it is a miserable time. Signs of teething include lots of finger or fist-chewing and dribbling, and can be accompanied by all sorts of other problems, such as nappy rash, diarrhoea, loss of appetite, eczema, spots, colds, fevers and ear problems. Teething puts stress on the immune system with the pain and inflammation of the gums.

They need plenty of comfort and things to bite on. Try to avoid using plastic teethers because of the risk of chemicals leaching from the plastic. Textured cloth like towelling or a suitable soft baby toy, a small wooden spoon or toy or traditional teething ring are all effective.

HERBS

- Chamomile and Limeflowers can help to calm a fractious baby, give regularly during the day while your baby is teething.
- Chamomile (Roman), Clove, Lavender or Myrrh essential oil – just 1 drop of a good quality oil in a little vegetable oil or honey can be rubbed onto the gum when teething pain is severe.
- See also page 74.

THREADWORMS

These are the most common type of worms and appear as pieces of white thread about 1cm long in the stools. Small children are particularly susceptible to picking up worms from dirty hands. Signs include anal itching, loss of weight, constipation or diarrhoea, tummy ache, bad breath, dark circles under the eyes, poor sleep, tiredness and irritability and frequent infections.

Adult threadworms do not live longer than 6 weeks and for the development of fresh worms, eggs must be swallowed and exposed to the action of the digestive system. In order to multiply adult worms lay their eggs around the anus at night which causes itching. Scratching the area allows eggs to be transmitted, via the hands if unwashed, to the mouth when eating or thumb sucking, or to the hands or food of others. Highly contagious, threadworms spread easily through the family and the school class without strict hygiene measures. Anthelmintics are effective, but need to be combined with hygiene measures to break the cycle of reinfection. Even when only one member of the family is affected all the members need treating. Each member of the family should be allocated their own towels and flannels which need to be kept separate and hot-washed regularly.

Teach children to wash their hands before eating, after each visit to the toilet and after playing outside or touching animals. Don't allow dogs to lick children's faces and ensure pets are free of worms. Discourage children from scratching an itchy bottom, keep finger nails short and try to scrub them with a nail brush daily. Close fitting pants worn at night and cotton gloves if necessary help prevent transfer – these should be changed daily and hot washed. A bath or shower in the morning will remove eggs laid during the night.

Not all children get worms while some are more susceptible than others. A healthy diet and regular bowel movements with no constipation will ensure a healthy digestive system and provide an unwelcome environment for worms to live in.

WHEN TO SEEK PROFESSIONAL ADVICE

- Seek the advice of a qualified Herbalist for correct treatment and dosage for babies and very young children.
- If there is resistance to treatment or repeated infestation. Anthelmintics are not for long-term use.

- If you suspect roundworm, or tapeworm which poses a serious risk to health.
- If you are pregnant – anthelmintics must not be used.

DIET

- Avoid sugar, especially refined sugars and carbohydrates and foods that contain them, for example breakfast cereals, cakes, biscuits, chocolate, drinks etc. Worms thrive in a sweet environment!
- Worm-repelling foods include onions and garlic, pumpkin seeds which can be ground up, apples and carrots eaten raw, grated or juiced, cabbage, pineapple, coconut, pomegranates, papaya and figs. These are best given on an empty stomach before breakfast. Live plain yoghurt helps to encourage a healthy gut flora and can be eaten daily, a pinch of cayenne might be added to this if your child is old enough to tolerate it. Alternatively, give Acidophilus powder as a supplement.

HERBS

- The herbs used to expel worms are very bitter to taste and best taken in capsule form, which is problematic when treating young children. Small liquid doses in heavy disguise or powders mixed with honey or molasses need to be used. Give the herbs for one week and repeat again one week later.
- Anthelmintics include Quassia, Tansy and Wormwood.
- Angelica, Centaury and Vervain are useful digestive herbs.
- Echinacea can be used to boost the immune system.
- Laxatives like Dandelion Root and Liquorice, especially if there is any constipation, speed up the expulsion of worms.
- 1-2 drops of Eucalyptus, Lavender or Tea Tree essential oil in ½ a tea-spoon of Garlic oil, Olive oil or Calendula (Marigold) ointment can be rubbed onto the anus at night to soothe itching and discourage worms from laying eggs.

THRUSH

Babies in particular are prone to this fungal infection. Oral thrush appears inside the mouth on the cheeks or tongue as white patches which are red underneath. It is also a common cause of nappy rash.

Treatment is dependent upon the age of the child. If a solely breast-fed baby, mum can take the herbs. Mum, in fact, might well be infecting/reinfecting baby and will need to treat her nipples after each feed. See also *Candida/Candidiasis.*

HERBS

- Marigold and Thyme can be given and also used as a wash on the affected areas.

- Tea Tree essential oil is an effective antifungal, this can be used as an oil in the bath or in a cream. If breastfeeding any residue of cream should be washed off before a feed.

TONSILLITIS

The tonsils comprise of lymphatic tissue in the throat where they protect the body from infection and potential allergens entering via the mouth and nose. They filter toxins from the respiratory system.

Tonsillitis describes the tonsils when they become inflamed, swollen and painful in response to an infection. They enlarge in order to increase their capabilities in dealing with the infection and prevent it going further into the body. For this reason the tonsils should be nurtured and problems seen as a warning sign. Surgical removal is a last resort.

Acute tonsillitis frequently accompanies a cold or flu virus, when the system is congested and overloaded with toxins. The child complains of a painful sore throat and the tonsils are red and swollen. The adenoids are usually also involved causing mouth breathing and snoring, while the swollen tonsils can block the eustachian tube and cause earache and/or infection.

The presence of pus on the tonsils suggests the infection is bacterial in which case the tonsillitis usually starts suddenly with a severe sore throat and swollen glands in the neck. This is often accompanied by a fever.

Chronic tonsillitis is where the tonsils remain swollen between bouts of recurrent tonsillitis. Repeated antibiotics usually compound the situation. Congestion in the system from poor digestion and elimination and chronic catarrh overwork the tonsils. There is frequently an intolerance to cow's milk or there may be an allergy. Environmental pollutants like cigarette smoke should be considered. There might also be an emotional element, the throat area being linked to the voice and the expression of feelings. These might be suppressed in children who find communicating their feelings difficult. See also *Adenoids, Allergies, Earache/Ear infections, Fever* and *Sore throat.*

WHEN TO SEEK PROFESSIONAL HELP

- Acute tonsillitis needs prompt, effective treatment. Streptococcal infection should be ruled out if the infection is bacterial.
- Chronic tonsillitis needs thorough investigation.

DIET

- See *Diet during infections* on page 19.
- Liquids like fruit and vegetable juices and soups will be easiest to swallow. Beetroot, carrots, blackcurrants and grapes are all beneficial.
- Remove milk products and sugar from the diet during the infection.
- Supplements of Garlic and Vitamin C can be given regularly while acute.
- Honey and lemon can be very soothing. One teaspoon of honey with the juice of ½ a lemon in hot water.

HERBS

- Myrrh, Rosemary and Sage can be used in a gargle or throat spray.
- Thyme is important as an antiseptic.
- Cleavers and Marigold are a must for lymphatic function.
- Compresses of the above can be applied externally to the throat area.
- Echinacea and Elderberry help boost the immune system and can be given every 2-3 hours while acute.
- Propolis products will help fight the infection and soothe the throat.
- Nebuliser oil (see page 40) can be applied to the chest and throat or used in a nebuliser or burner.

VERRUCAS

See *Warts* and *Verrucas*.

VIRAL INFECTIONS

There are numerous viral infections that have no specific title, alongside ones like Hand, Foot and Mouth and Slap cheek (Erythema). Treat the symptoms as above for Fever etc.

WARTS *and* VERRUCAS

Warts are caused by a virus which causes an excess of skin growth. When they appear on the foot they are called verrucas and grow inwards, which can cause discomfort if they become large. They are slightly contagious.

HERBS

- Boost the immune system with Echinacea.
- The most effective external applications are the fresh, milky sap of Dandelion or the yellow latex of Celandine. Otherwise tinctures of these can be used.
- Thuja (Tree of Life) can be given as tincture 10 drops twice a day for 4-8 weeks.
- Tea Tree essential oil can be applied neat.

WORMS

See *Threadworms*.

WHOOPING COUGH

This is a contagious childhood illness caused by the Bordetella pertussis bacteria which occurs most commonly in the under 10's. The incubation period is 7-14 days until the catarrhal stage. This stage is highly infectious and is accompanied by a runny nose, conjuctivitis and an unproductive cough. It is almost impossible to diagnose during this very contagious stage. After about a week, however, there are severe coughing bouts (the paroxysmal stage), usually at night, which end in the characteristic whoop, and perhaps vomiting. In older children and adults the air passages are wider and the whoop is usually absent. The paroxysmal stage can last a couple of weeks, with symptoms gradually declining over the subsequent few weeks, but the cough can persist for much longer.

It is the very young who are most at risk, especially the newborn, whose air passages are narrow and lungs immature. Congestion and coughing can seriously diminish the oxygen supply to the brain, causing convulsions. Serious consequences are more likely if your child's health has been previously compromised. It is wise to avoid unneccessary exposure to coughs and colds with very young babies.

The most important thing is to treat any cough or cold when it first appears by cutting out dairy products, boosting the immune system and giving herbs for the respiratory system.

Vaccination does not mean your child will not get whooping cough. See also *Anxiety, Colds* and *Coughs*.

WHEN TO SEEK PROFESSIONAL ADVICE

- Whooping cough is a notifiable disease so contact your GP as well as a qualified Herbalist.

DIET

- See *Diet during infections* on page 19.
- Vomiting can lead to loss of weight. Give small meals regularly, or give the main meal earlier in the day if it is the coughing bouts at night that lead to vomiting. Make sure your child is relaxed and the environment calm at meal times.

HERBS

- Elecampane, Sundew and Thyme are antiseptic, antispasmodic and expectorant.

- Wild Cherry Bark has a sedative effect on the cough reflex and can be used during the paroxysmal stage.

- Herbs will need to be given every 1–2 hours when the symptoms are severe.

- Use herbs like Chamomile, Lemon Balm and Limeflowers to relax and relieve anxiety.

- Use Nebuliser oil (see page 40) on the chest and in inhalations and vaporisers.

- Use Bach Flower Rescue Remedy for fear and panic.

- If Whooping cough is in your area, or your child has been in contact with an infected child give precautionary measures such as Echinacea, Elderberry, Coltsfoot and Hyssop everyday. Use Thyme and Propolis as a mouth and throat spray.

9 | A basic dispensary for children

The herbs given below are an idea of some basic herbs you will need to have on hand. You can simply add to them according to your family's needs.

Herbs

For internal use:

- Chamomile – soothing and calming, for digestive upsets, sleeplessness.
- Echinacea tincture – boosts the immune system, use for viral and bacterial infections.
- Elderflowers – colds, catarrh, sore throat, fever.
- Limeflowers – relaxing, fever.
- Thyme tincture or syrup – coughs.
- Liquorice tincture – a small amount improves the flavour of strong tasting medicines and is soothing to coughs, helps keep the bowels moving during illnesses.
- Elderberry tincture – give during the winter months to increase resistance to bugs. It also tastes good!

For external use:

- Arnica – bruises, sprains – tincture/cream.
- Marigold (Calendula) – eyebath for conjuctivitis, antiseptic first aid remedy for cuts and abrasions, nappy rash – tincture/cream.
- St John's Wort oil – earache, burns, nappy rash.
- Distilled Witch Hazel – bumps and bruises, soothes irritated skin.
- Healing cream – a mixture of Comfrey, Marigold, Lavender essential oil, St John's Wort oil and Witch Hazel can be used on any skin problem.

Essential oils

- Eucalyptus – coughs and colds.
- Lavender – burns, cuts, earache.
- Tea tree – athlete's foot, thrush/fungal infections.

Other natural remedies

- Bach Flower Rescue Remedy.
- Homoeopathic Arnica.

10 | Herbal first aid

Herbs work remarkably well in acute situations. Of course, a first aid course is invaluable backup in emergency situations.

Bites and Stings

- Citronella, Eucalyptus, Lavender, Lemon Grass, Rosemary or Tea Tree essential oil can be placed in a dish and kept next to the bed at night or used in an oil burner to repel insects. Alternatively, use a couple of drops on a handkerchief or applied to clothing.

- Feverfew or Neem can be used externally in a lotion or spray and applied to the skin as a repellent.

- Feverfew tincture can be given internally as an effective repellent, but needs to be taken consistently on a daily basis. For children (and adults) who are sensitive to insect bites and those insects find particularly attractive give 2-10 drops twice a day.

- Rue, Rosemary, Tansy, Southernwood and Wormwood can be hung in rooms as a natural insect repellent.

- For bites apply a mixture of tinctures of Arnica, Burdock, Echinacea, Feverfew, Nettle and Yellow Dock. (NB Arnica should not be used on broken skin).

- Lavender or Tea Tree essential oil can be applied neat to bites.

- Apply vinegar to wasp and jelly fish stings and a solution of bicarbonate of soda to bee stings.

Burns

- Put the area under cold water immediately and keep it there for several minutes.

- Apply St John's Wort oil, Lavender essential oil, Aloe gel or Marigold (Calendula) cream.

- Use Healing cream (see *Cuts and Grazes*).
- Severe burns need hospital treatment.

Bruises
- Apply Arnica, Horsechestnut or Witch Hazel.
- Use Comfrey or Healing cream (see *Cuts and Grazes*) for bad bruises.

Cuts and Grazes
- Clean area with diluted tincture of calendula, myrrh or golden seal.
- Apply Healing cream made up of Comfrey, Lavender essential oil, Marigold, St. John's Wort oil and Witch Hazel.

Nose bleeds
- Seek medical attention if the nosebleed follows a blow to the head.
- Apply cold compresses of witch hazel or yarrow over the bridge of the nose.

Shock
- Give Bach Flower Rescue Remedy.
- Soothing teas of Chamomile, Lemon Balm and Limeflowers will calm.
- Homoeopathic Arnica can be given.

Splinters
- Stubborn splinters can be drawn out with a drawing cream made up of Marshmallow Root and Slippery Elm powders in an aqueous base cream.
- Essential oils of Lavender or Tea tree and Myrrh tincture or essential oil can be added to make the cream antiseptic.

Sprains
- After applying ice, cold water or witch hazel use arnica cream.
- Comfrey Leaf internally and Comfrey cream, ideally with cayenne added to increase blood flow to the area, externally will help speed healing.
- If nothing else is available bruise a cabbage leaf and wrap this over the area.

Sunburn

- Liberally apply Aloe Vera gel to cool.
- Apply St John's Wort oil with Lavender essential oil or Healing cream (see *Cuts and Grazes*).
- Distilled Witch Hazel is cooling and soothing.
- Use Lemon juice if you have nothing else to hand.

Teething pain / Toothache

- Pure German or Roman Chamomile essential oil – dilute one drop in ½ to 1 tsp of vegetable oil and rub some onto the gum with a finger.
- Clove essential oil is a traditional and stronger painkiller – dilute as for Chamomile oil.
- Give Chamomile tea to calm or Homoeopathic Chamomilla as tablets or granules.
- New Era tissue salts for Infants Teething Pains can be used daily to alleviate the discomfort.

Travel sickness

- Ginger taken 10–30 minutes before travel either as 2–10 drops of tincture or 1–2 capsules.
- Seabands worn like sweatbands on the wrists apply pressure to acupuncture points used to alleviate nausea.

11 | Further reading

The Herbal for Mother and Child by Anne McIntyre, Element.

Herbal First Aid by Andrew Chevallier, Amberwood.

Vaccinations: A Thoughtful Parent's Guide by Aviva Jill Romm, Healing Arts Press, Vermont.

What Really Works for Kids by Susan Clark, Bantam Press.

11 | Useful addresses

The National Institute of Medical Herbalists
56 Longbrook Street, Exeter EX4 6AH
Tel: 01392 426022

The Informed Parent
PO Box 870, Harrow, Middlesex HA3 7UW
Tel/Fax: 020 8861 1022
www.informedparent.co.uk

HERBAL DISPENSARIES

Aquitaine Apothecary
119 High Street, Sevenoaks, Kent TN13 1XR
Tel: 01732 749789

Baldwins
171-173 Walworth Road, London SE17 1RW
Tel: 0207 7035550

Bio-Health Ltd *(Herbal Medicine manufacturers)*
Culpeper Close, Medway City Estate, Rochester, Kent ME2 4HU
Tel: 01634 290115

Gaia Herbal Apothecary
London Road, Forest Row, East Sussex RH18 5EZ
Tel: 01342 822716

Hambly's Herbal Dispensary
The Old Dairy, Durgates, Wadhurst, East Sussex TN5 6DE
Tel: 01892 783027
www.hamblys.net

Herbs for Health
1 Otago Terrace, St Saviours Road, Larkhall, Bath, Avon BA1 6SX
Tel: 01225 427999

Napiers Dispensary
18 Bristo Place, Edinburgh EH1 1EZ
Tel: 0131 225 5542

Nature's Dispensary
7 Mill street, Oakham, Rutland LE15 6EA
Tel: 01572 771231

Ralph and Evans
8 West Street, West Malling, Kent ME19 6QX
Tel: 01732 871818
& 11 Best Lane, Canterbury, Kent CT1 2 JB
Tel: 01227 471771

The Natural Health Care Centre & Herbal Dispensary
Ty Clyd, Long Street, Newport, Dyfed SA42 0TL
Tel: 01239 820050

OTHER BOOKS from AMBERWOOD PUBLISHING:

AROMATHERAPY

Aromatherapy – A Guide for Home Use by Christine Westwood. £1.99.
Aromatherapy – For Stress Management by Christine Westwood. £3.50.
Aromatherapy – For Healthy Legs and Feet by Christine Westwood. £2.99.
Aromatherapy – A Nurses Guide by Ann Percival. £3.50.
Aromatherapy – A Nurses Guide for Women by Ann Percival. £2.99.
Aromatherapy – Simply For You by Marion Del Gaudio Mak. £2.99.
Aroma Science – The Chemistry & Bioactivity of Essential Oils by Dr Maria Lis-Balchin. £5.99.
Aromatherapy – Essential Oils in Colour by Dr. Rosemary Caddy. £9.99.
Aromatherapy – The Essential Blending Guide by Dr. Rosemary Caddy. £12.99
Aromatherapy Lexicon – The Essential Reference by Geoff Lyth and Sue Charles. £4.99.
Aromatherapy – The Baby Book by Marion Del Gaudio Mak. £3.99
Aromatherapy – The Pregnancy Book by Jennie Supper. £5.99

HERBAL

Ginkgo Biloba – Ancient Medicine by Dr Desmond Corrigan. £2.99.
Echinacea – Indian Medicine for the Immune System by Dr Desmond Corrigan. £2.99.
Herbal Medicine for Sleep & Relaxation by Dr Desmond Corrigan. £2.99.
Garlic– How Garlic Protects Your Heart by Prof E. Ernst. £3.99.
Phytotherapy – Fifty Vital Herbs by Andrew Chevallier. £6.99
Natural Taste – Herbal Teas, A Guide for Home Use by Andrew Chevallier. £3.50.
Woman Medicine – Vitex Agnus Castus by Simon Mills. £2.99.
Menopause – The Herbal Way by Andrew Chevallier. £5.99
Herbal First Aid – Natural Medicine by Andrew Chevallier. £3.50.
Plant Medicine – A Guide for Home Use by Charlotte Mitchell. £2.99.
Cancer – Herbs in Holistic Healthcare by Dr J. Walker. £15.99.

GENERAL HEALTHCARE

Insomnia – Doctor I Can't Sleep by Dr Adrian Williams. £2.99.
Eyecare Eyewear – For Better Vision by Mark Rossi. £3.99.
Arthritis and Rheumatism – The Sufferers Guide by Dr John Cosh. £4.95.
Feng Shui – A Guide for Home Use by Karen Ward. £2.99

NUTRITION

Causes & Prevention of Vitamin Deficiency by Dr L. Mervyn. £2.99
Vitamins ABC and Other Food Facts (for Children) by E. Palmer. £3.99
All You Ever Wanted To Know About Vitamins by Dr Leonard Mervyn. £6.99.

CALL FOR INFORMATION: **(01634) 290115** or
email: **info@amberwoodpublishing.com** *www:* **amberwoodpublishing.com**